More than Just Medicine

Exploring Alternative Medicine

Paolo Jose de Luna

held against the publisher for any reparation, damages, or monetary loss due to the information herein, either directly or indirectly.

The information herein is offered for informational purposes solely and is universal as so. The presentation of the information is without a contract or any type of guarantee. The trademarks that are used are without any consent, and the publication of the trademark is without permission or backing by the trademark owner. All trademarks and brands within this book are for clarifying purposes only and are owned by the owners themselves, not affiliated with this document.

Table of Contents

Introduction

Over the years, researchers have conducted all kinds of studies to benefit the healthcare industry. Without a doubt, this field has attracted a lot of investment from stakeholders who are interested in finding the most effective ways to prevent, manage, and cure a wide range of health problems that are experienced by people across the world. However, researchers are yet to find answers to some of the most pressing problems that have not been solved. For this reason, humans are eager to find solutions to things that have been unsolved.

Today, patients have access to a wide selection of medications, surgical procedures, diagnostic examinations, and laboratory tests. This is possible because the healthcare sector has evolved in various dimensions. New discoveries and technological advancements have revolutionized everything and contributed to the development of today's sophisticated healthcare practices.

Besides the introduction of better health practices and new methods of curing health problems and improving people's lives, one of the key changes that have taken place is the establishment of reliable sources of knowledge in the healthcare industry. This knowledge has always been and will be shared across generations. Thanks to this practice of passing knowledge from generation to generation, humans have been able to learn from their predecessors and even acquire more knowledge by doing more research.

Although scientific research has played a significant role in providing more knowledge and improving healthcare practices, the entire field of healthcare is not based on science. For many years, humans have learned how to use other options to improve their lives. There are different types of therapeutic techniques used to address a wide range of health problems. For many years, humans have been able to prevent, manage, and treat many health problems without using medications and procedures that are based on scientific research and evidence.

Many people around the world are aware of the potential benefits of the different types of alternative medicine. These treatment options have provided us with alternative methods as well as new possibilities for disease prevention, treatment, and wellness. Nowadays, it is possible to improve our health and overall well-being without using modern medications and procedures that are found in clinical settings.

Alternative medicine is almost everywhere, and people across the world appreciate its health benefits. Of course, contemporary medicine provides us with a variety of drugs that can alleviate the symptoms of different types of diseases. However, these drugs usually cause adverse reactions and side effects. The truth of the matter is that drug manufacturers usually combine different types of chemicals that may interfere with the body's normal functions. Once ingested, these chemicals are basically foreign substances in the human body. For this reason, patients can expect to experience side effects or adverse reactions when using manufactured drugs.

The good news is that humans have discovered and learned to utilize alternative medicine for many health problems that are experienced today. Alternative medicine usually involves the use of natural methods to improve an individual's health and promote wellness. With this type of medicine, patients are able to treat diseases and promote their overall well-being without relying on the usual drugs and surgical procedures. Generally, alternative medicine is about utilizing natural methods to prevent, manage and treat health problems.

Based on the available evidence, alternative medicine has become popular in the modern healthcare industry with many people using it to cure a number of health problems. However, some people are yet to be convinced that alternative medicine can be a great option for those looking for effective treatment methods. They have the right to express their skepticism because there are all kinds of scams claiming to be the latest and most effective solutions to a wide range of health problems.

With that in mind, you must be cautious at all times. It would help to do further research or seek advice from a health expert with regard to the kind of treatment that you wish to have. Generally, the choice is all yours and the most important thing is to choose options that are safe and known effective.

CHAPTER 1:

Alternative Medicine Explained

If you haven't heard of or used any form of alternative medicine before, don't worry because you are about to learn what it's all about. In simple terms, alternative medicine refers to the practice of using natural remedies or methods to promote an individual's health and overall wellbeing. The main difference between conventional medicine and alternative medicine is that the former mainly involves the use of drugs and surgical procedures while the latter involves the use of natural remedies.

The practice of alternative medicine encompasses different types of healing techniques that are used to improve one's health. Unlike conventional medicine, alternative medicine does not rely on evidence to support its benefits. However, many health advocates have studied alternative medicine for many years to learn about its potential uses and benefits.

With influence from our ancestors and significant developments that have taken place over time, alternative medicine has become an important part of the modern-day healthcare practice. It's now a good option for people who believe in natural methods of preventing and treating the health problems they experience. Generally, alternative medicine is gaining popularity in today's healthcare industry and has been accepted by scientists and healthcare practitioners. In fact, many people from different parts of the world use one or several types of alternative medicine to address everyday health problems and improve their lives.

Alternative medicine includes a broad range of practices. It's more than just promoting the use of natural ways to improve human health. One of the key developments in the healthcare sector in recent years is the use of alternative medicine practices together with modern medicine. Modern medicine is combined with alternative medicine based on beliefs, rather than scientific evidence, to form what is commonly known as "*complementary medicine*". However, when conventional medicine is combined with alternative medicine based on scientific evidence, we get what is known as "*integrated medicine*".

As you can see, alternative medicine has transformed the healthcare industry because it can work with other types of medicine with or without scientific evidence. This means that people with different types of health problems can benefit from a variety of treatment options that incorporate purely natural means or natural means combined with manufactured drugs.

People who are skeptical about alternative medicine are usually afraid of unproven healing practices that may appear unusual. They are also afraid of the hoaxes associated with these practices. However, the truth is that alternative medicine presents a number of health benefits to patients with different types of health conditions. Additionally, alternative medicine comes from natural sources and involves the use of safe organic methods to heal without relying on chemical-based drugs.

Alternative medicine is also associated with certain economic benefits when it comes to the costs of treatment. If you've used conventional medicine at some point, you know that you can pay huge sums of money depending on how serious your health condition is. Alternative medicine reduces the costs associated with treatment because patients are not required to purchase expensive drugs. It's a great option if you have limited financial resources.

However, it's important to take the necessary precautions when using any form of alternative medicine. The truth of the matter is that most of them, especially the most recent ones, lack scientific evidence. It may be difficult to provide evidence to support the claim that certain types of alternative medicine have significant benefits when ingested or used for health purposes. Before you decide to use alternative medicine, make sure you have sufficient information regarding its benefits.

If you choose to take any kind of alternative medicine, you can expect to come across practices that are somewhat hard to believe. In this book, we will mainly focus on alternative medicine practices that have been found to be effective in treating certain health conditions. We will let you know the supporting evidence based on research studies so you can know which options choose. The options discussed here have a wide range of benefits including physical and psychological benefits. Some of them even have spiritual benefits if you are a spiritual person.

CHAPTER 2:
When Did Alternative Medicine Start?

Humans have used a variety of alternative medicine for a very long time. The use of alternative medicine can be traced back to thousands of years ago. However, we may not be able to tell the exact time when humans started to use alternative medicine. One of the reasons why this is difficult is because the practice involves a wide range of health practices that didn't start at the same time.

There are different stories about the origin of alternative medicine. For instance, there are speculations that humans started to use alternative medicine in the prehistoric period. During this era, our ancestors would continually improvise healthcare practices to provide better healthcare services to the sick. It's also believed that cavemen used traditional methods to treat injuries and even cure illnesses during the Stone Age years. They relied on natural remedies from different types of plants and herbs to treat wounds and relieve various symptoms. It's also believed that cavemen used fire to close wounds. Another fascinating practice during the era of cavemen was the use of makeshift treatment methods to help those suffering from mental problems.

One of the notable eras in the history of alternative medicine was the era of the ancient Chinese. The Chinese people played a very important role in the development of various treatment methods that have built the practice of alternative medicine. The Chinese are actually known for their extensive use of herbal remedies that are an important part of today's alternative medicine. Over the years, Chinese herbal remedies have been incorporated into various healthcare practices and contributed to the development of what is known as conventional medicine today. Traditional Chinese herbal medicine is characterized by different types of mixtures, potions or elixirs that contain various herbs and oils with the power to relieve the symptoms of different health conditions.

Overall, Asian countries have played a vital role in popularizing alternative medicine. They are famous for contributing to the development and advancement of alternative healthcare practices that are believed to control the flow of energy or *chi* in the human body. Some of the widely used forms of alternative medicine with an Asian origin include acupuncture, Ayurvedic medicine, and meditation.

Although alternative medicine has been around for thousands of years, the practice started to gain popularity during the nineteenth century. In the 1970s, healthcare providers didn't consider alternative medicine practitioners as members of the medical community. In fact, alternative medicine practitioners were considered to be quack doctors because they neither had knowledge-based principles nor scientific evidence to prove that their type of medicine worked.

Medical practitioners who used conventional medicine were more interested in medical practices with scientific evidence. For this reason, alternative medicine practitioners were rejected by those who believed in conventional medicine. Members of the medical community regarded alternative health practices as a serious health risk.

However, it's important to note that conventional medicine also posed certain health risks at that time. For example, medical doctors risked the lives of patients by treating them without sufficient assessment data. Patients would undergo unsafe surgical procedures such as lobotomy without proper assessments. In addition to the lack of reliable assessment data, medical doctors performed some surgical procedures without taking the necessary precautions. Most surgical procedures involved the use of alcohol because it was the most popular anesthetic. Patients would undergo medical procedures without a reliable anesthetic. Another significant problem was the lack of reliable antibiotics for preventing infections. The point is that conventional medicine had its own drawbacks despite having scientific evidence.

One of the key figures in the history of alternative medicine is an American politician, author, and attorney called Tom Harkin. Since 1991, he has been influential in promoting the use of alternative medicine. One of the recommendable things he did for the alternative medicine industry was to provide funds. To show his passion for alternative medicine, Harkin gave 2 million dollars to the Office of the Study of Unconventional Medical Practices (OSUMP), which is now known as the National

Center for Complementary and Integrative Health (NCCIH).

Before it received its current name, the NCCIH was renamed from OSUMP to the Office of Alternative Medicine (OAM) and the National Center for Complementary and Alternative Medicine (NCCAM). When working as the OAM, the NCCIH collaborated with the National Institute of Health (NIH) to find scientific evidence to support the practice of alternative medicine. They wanted the public to know whether alternative medicine was beneficial or harmful.

Since then, many people started to recognize the potential benefits of alternative medicine. By 1993, alternative medicine was already popular in Great Britain capturing the attention of prominent figures like Prince Charles himself. Yes, the prince believed in the healing powers of alternative medicine practices such as homeopathy. He claimed that such practices were effective and decided to establish the Foundation for Integrated Health (FIH). The foundation was established for the purposes of studying and exploring safe practices for alternative medicine practitioners. It would help to integrate alternative medicine with conventional medicine. The FIH was approved almost immediately and received monetary support from the government of Britain through the Department of Health.

Alternative medicine is now popular thanks to the amount of support received from various stakeholder including practitioners, politicians, scientists, patients and the society at large. Alternative medicine is now practiced all over the world because of this support and many people have benefited from it in different ways. People are using it on a daily basis to address a variety of health issues without using conventional drugs.

However, there is a significant gap regarding the evidence needed to help people recognize alternative medicine as an effective and safe method of preventing and treating certain health conditions. For this reason, more research is needed to provide enough evidence to people who are still skeptical about the different types of alternative medicine that are used today.

When choosing the appropriate form of alternative medicine, it's important to keep in mind that there are people who claim to introduce new forms of alternative medicine only to paint a negative image of alternative medicine. Some of them are busy promoting ineffective practices that are just hoaxes. You should stay away from such people, so you need to be careful if you decide to use any form of alternative medicine. Of course, you don't want to waste your time and money on ineffective health practices that might harm your body.

Make sure the selected options are efficient and safe before you ingest or apply on your body.

CHAPTER 3:

Types of Alternative Medicine

So far, we've learned what alternative medicine is and explored its history. Now that you know where this type of medicine came from, the next step is to explore the various options for those looking for effective alternative medicines. Alternative medicine involves different practices that will be discussed in this section of the book. Looking at the history of alternative medicine, there is no doubt that the practice has evolved over the years.

Today, those willing to try alternative medicine can choose from a wide range of different practices that humans have utilized and perfected for many years. As you look for your favorite, remember some of them may have significant health benefits while others may not have proven health benefits. Let's talk about some popular options for alternative medicine enthusiasts.

Acupuncture

As mentioned earlier, the Chinese are among
the key pioneers of alternative medicine. They
are famous for a variety of traditional health
practices that have lasted thousands of years.
Acupuncture is one of the most popular types of
alternative medicine based on the health
practices of ancient Chinese people. During an
acupuncture session, the practitioner inserts
needles into various pressure points to
manipulate energy flow in the patient's body.
It's believed that this method of treatment has
the power to improve the patient's health by
changing or blocking energy flow.

People who practice acupuncture also believe
that the same health effects can be achieved by
applying pressure, lasers or heat on the various
pressure points. The practitioner needs to know
the exact areas to apply pressure and know how
to insert the needs without hurting the patient.
This practice may look unusual if you've never

done or seen it, but many people have benefited from it. It still exists because people have seen and experienced its health benefits.

According to information from various sources, the first form of acupuncture was practiced in China around 100 B.C. At that time, those who practiced acupuncture would manipulate the *yin* (negative) and *yang* (positive) energies. Acupuncture also involved studying celestial and lunar bodies. However, there was a significant decrease in the number of people who practiced acupuncture in China. The practice eventually became less popular in China and was replaced by the widely accepted practice of herbal medicine. However, this did not prevent acupuncture from spreading to other parts of the world. The practice spread to other regions starting with several Asian countries including India, Japan, and Vietnam.

After reaching Asian nations, acupuncture also spread to the United States of America and was already popular in the 1990s. It also gained popularity in other western nations. By the time the practice reached western countries, a number of significant changes had taken place. It was more than a health practice based on traditional Chinese health practices. Many years later, humans were able to identify scientific evidence to support the benefits of acupuncture as claimed by people who used this form of alternative medicine to treat the sick and improve people's health. Today, some people still practice acupuncture because of the available evidence of its effectiveness in treating certain health conditions.

People who believe in the healing power of acupuncture use it to treat a variety of health conditions including different types of pains and body aches. Many of the people who use this type of alternative medicine are those suffering back pain. In addition to helping people with pains and aches, acupuncture is considered to be an effective treatment for some common health conditions.

When it comes to the actual treatment process, acupuncture is usually combined with conventional medicine and used as a form of therapy. It is also combined with other alternative medicines in order to achieve the best results. Generally, you'll rarely find an acupuncture practitioner who uses the needles alone without administering some form of conventional medicine.

Of course, people who are skeptical about alternative health practices like acupuncture may want to know if scientific research supports this type of medicine. Researches have conducted different types of studies that have produced positive results. Some research findings have revealed that patients suffering from certain health conditions may benefit from acupuncture. From a clinical perspective, the practice of acupuncture revolves around body pauses and heat. The first step of a typical acupuncture process involves evaluating your body to check your pulse. Sometimes the practitioner may inspect your tongue before the session begins. The initial evaluation may last for minutes or an hour depending on the type of evaluation the practitioner wants to do.

Benefits of Acupuncture

Acupuncture offers a wide range of health benefits including the power to:

- Relieve the pain caused by migraines and headaches
- Promote better sleeping patterns
- Improve mood
- Help hypertensive patients by reducing blood pressure
- Reduce stress levels
- Relieve symptoms of insomnia
- Lower the frequency and severity of hot flashes during menopause
- Improve the body's immune system
- Reduce the effects of allergies

- Reduce the risk of developing GERD or gastroesophageal reflux disease
- Reduce the effects of heartburn
- Improve functions of the digestive system
- Prevent the development of infections
- Relieve back pain
- Help overweight people during the weight loss process

Acupressure

Acupressure is another type of alternative medicine with roots in traditional Chinese medicine. This treatment method has been around for thousands of years and is based on the same principles as acupuncture. The main difference is that acupressure does not involve the use of needles. People who practice acupressure use their fingers to press key points that stimulate the body's self-healing capabilities. This healing art is used to promote relaxation, treat diseases, and promote wellness.

According to traditional Chinese medical theory, the human body has special pressure points or acupressure points that lie along meridians. These are the same pressure point targeted when using acupuncture. It's believed that vital energy or *chi* flows through these channels. Sickness occurs as a result of a blockage or an imbalance within these meridians. Just like acupuncture, the practice of acupressure is thought to restore balance and promote health. In addition, acupressure is used to regulate opposing forces of negative energy (*yin*) and positive energy (*yang*). Generally, acupressure is used to correct functional imbalances and restores the flow of vital energy to help the body return to its natural state of wellbeing.

During an acupressure session, practitioners may use their fingers, palms, elbows, feet or special devices to gently press pressure points on the meridians. In addition to applying pressure, the practice of acupressure may involve massaging and stretching. Acupressure sessions usually take about an hour. Several acupressure sessions may be required in order to achieve the best results.

Benefits of Acupressure

Acupressure is believed to have the power to:
- Relieve stress-related health problems
- Promote deep relaxation

- Boost the functions of the immune system
- Reduce muscular tension in different parts of the body. For instance, self-acupressure is used to relieve back pain. It relaxes and tones the back muscles to make spinal adjustments more effective.
- Reduce physical and emotional pain
- Helps with blood circulation
- Break addictions by releasing stress, tension, and pain
- Boost sexual energy in lovemaking – Lovers can use full body embraces, touch, and kisses to released blocked sexual energy
- Treat specific health conditions such as chronic muscular pain, learning disorders, trauma, chronic fatigue, depression, anxiety, arthritis, headache, nausea, and fibromyalgia.
- Promote beauty – Acupressure beauty treatment methods enhance the tone of

facial muscles. In addition, acupressure is combined with facial exercises to relax the muscles, relieve congested areas, and release toxins. This improves your looks as well as how you feel.

Drawbacks of Acupressure

- Pressing the wrong points may not relieve the problem
- Too much pressure may cause problems especially during pregnancy
- Acupressure does not cure serious health problems such as heart and kidney disease
- It may consume a lot of time
- Some symptoms will only disappear for a short period

Herbal Medicine

Herbal medicine is a health practice that involves the use of naturally occurring, plant-based remedies to treat ailments and promote health. It is among the oldest and most extensive forms of alternative medicine you'll find today. Herbal medicine is usually a combination of different plant-based substances with the power to treat various health problems. People who practice herbal medicine have access to a wide selection of herbs as well as spices from all regions of the world. This means that users have plenty of options depending on the ingredients they prefer and where they live. Depending on the herbs used, herbal medicine can treat common ailments as well as more serious health problems. Basically, you may be able to relieve certain health problems at home if you can find the right ingredients.

In addition to the power to treat a number of health conditions, herbal medicine is popular around the world for various reasons. First, we've mentioned that there are thousands of options when it comes to herbs for preparing herbal medicine, so people love it because of variety. Second, many of the studies focusing on herbal medicine have revealed that this form of alternative medicine is effective in treating certain health problems. Today, many health care practitioners and scientists recommended it to patients suffering from ailments that can be cured using herbs.

Nowadays, it's not surprising to come across all kinds of herbal medicines as well as supplements when you visit your local market. Chances are you'll find some in the nearest local drugstore. Your physician may even decide to prescribe herbal medicines that have been proven to be an effective cure for your health condition. If you are looking for alternative medicine, the good news is that you can expect to find herbal medicine everywhere.

Benefits of Herbal Medicine

- One of the reasons why herbal medicine is a good option is that the chances of experiencing adverse reactions and side effects are very low. If you use chemical-based drugs, you are more likely to experience side effects compared to someone who uses herbal medicines.

- Another benefit of using herbal medicine is that it comes from natural sources and uses an organic approach. This means that herbal medicine is a healthier and safer option, unlike manufactured medicines.

- Herbal medicine is a great option for people with chronic health problems such as hypertension, diabetes, and cancer. Most herbal remedies contain powerful antioxidants that play a vital role in fighting free radicals that damage body cells. Therefore, herbal remedies can protect human body cells from damage and thus benefit those suffering from chronic health problems.

- The low cost of herbal medicine is another reason why people love this type of alternative medicine. Patients usually spend a lot of money on commercial drugs depending on the health problem they want to treat. Luckily, some of the health problems that require expensive drugs can be cured using affordable herbal medicines. Generally, herbal medicines tend to be more economical for many people.

- Availability is always an important factor to consider when looking for medicines. One of the best things about herbal medicines is that they are easy to find. You can prepare some varieties at home or buy them at the nearest drugstore.

As you can see, people suffering from certain health problems including chronic conditions can benefit from herbal medicine in different ways. It's not surprising to know that many people are more than willing to try this form of alternative medicine without being skeptical. In fact, many people are already using herbal medicines and adding herbal supplements to their diet plans.

Since herbal medicine is widely recommended by health practitioners, it has attracted the attention of many people who are looking for healthier and effective treatment options for various health conditions. Many people can afford it, so it will continue to be an important part of people's treatment and diet plans. You can't afford to claim that herbal medicine is a hoax because there's sufficient scientific evidence to prove the effectiveness of this type of medicine. The findings of many studies have shown that there are many effective herbal remedies for various ailments, so there's no need to be skeptical when taking herbal medicines.

Drawbacks of Herbal Medicine

Although herbal medicine offers many benefits, it also faces a number of challenges. It's important to know some of the drawbacks of this form of alternative medicine before you make a choice. Here are the negative aspects of some of the herbal medicines you'll find today:

- There are different types of health conditions with different signs and symptoms that cannot be relieved using certain herbal remedies. The plants, herbs and spices used to prepare herbal medicine have different qualities and may not be good for every health problem.

- The second problem associated with herbal medicine is to find the correct dosage. Herbal medicine is easy to prepare or find if you want to purchase, but you may have difficulty finding the correct dosage. This is especially true if you prepare your own herbal medicine at home. You may not know how much you need to take each day and how often you should take it.

- When taking herbal medicine, you may have to consult a physician if you are taking other drugs. This is important because some herbal medicines may cause adverse effects if they interact with certain drugs.

- Another significant challenge associated with the use of herbal remedies is that you may develop allergic reactions if you use medications with certain herbs. For this reason, it's advisable to pay attention to the plants, herbs or spices used to prepare the herbal medications and supplements you intend to take.

Chiropractic Medicine

Chiropractic medicine is another popular and effective type of alternative medicine with a wide range of benefits. The main goal of this form of treatment is to establish the diagnosis and cure for various health problems that affect specific parts of the human body. The key areas of focus include the body's skeletal system and the muscular system. Chiropractic medicine is particularly a good option for those suffering from back pain.

The theory behind chiropractic medicine is that different types of health problems that affect human health occur because of changes that interfere with our nervous system. The practice of chiropractic medicine involves manipulating the spine to make adjustments that can benefit the nervous system.

Many people in different parts of the world have found chiropractic medicine to be an effective method of treatment. As a result, this type of medicine is now among the widely used health practices by people who believe in the healing power of alternative medicine. One of the key things you'll notice about chiropractic medicine practitioners or chiropractors is that they are similar to health care providers in various ways.

Although chiropractic medicine mainly involves manipulating the spine, joint movements, and muscle exercises, it is similar to the usual healthcare services because it may include some form of counseling. For instance, chiropractors may offer life or health counseling services during a treatment session depending on what they think the patient needs.

Chiropractic medicine is basically about manipulating and aligning the spine. It's believed that this method of treatment improves an individual's overall health if the spine is properly aligned. If you choose this form of alternative medicine, you give the chiropractor permission to manipulate your spine and probably use other types of alternative medicine to promote your overall health and wellbeing. People who practice chiropractic medicine believe that the body heals to its optimum capacity when the spine and joints are aligned.

In most cases, people use chiropractic medicine to manipulate restricted joints. This includes joints restricted by various problems such as injuries from physical trauma, tear damage, and falls. In addition to relieving spinal pain, chiropractic medicine can be used to relieve pain in other parts of the body. It can be a great option if you are suffering from muscle, bone, tissue or joint pain. The best results can be achieved by combining chiropractic medicine with conventional medicine. Therefore, it's important to know which types of conventional medicine are effective in treating your health condition when combined with chiropractic medicine. You may need help from a physician.

Benefits of Chiropractic Medicine

Chiropractic medicine offers a number of benefits including the capability to:

- Relieve pain in different parts of the body including the back, joints, and the neck. Chiropractic medicine is also good for those suffering from bone and muscle pain. It can also be helpful if you are having headaches.
- Improve joint movement
- Lower blood pressure for people with hypertension
- Reduce damaging for people with whiplash
- Heal damaged body tissues

Drawbacks of Chiropractic Medicine

Chiropractic methods and other health practices that involve manipulating the body's spine are generally considered to be safe. They are also effective treatment options for those suffering from back and joint pain. However, it's important to note that any health practice that involves manipulating the spine may cause some contraindications. In fact, you could worsen your problem if you decide to use chiropractic medicine while suffering from a serious health condition. It would be better to ask your health practitioner before you take chiropractic treatment.

Here are some of the possible drawbacks of using chiropractic medicine:

- In some cases, chiropractors come across people who have suffered from spinal problems such as injuries. Other patients have tumors and other spinal abnormalities. People with such problems are advised to avoid chiropractic medicine to lower the risk of worsening their situation.

- There are also patients who come to the chiropractor with brittle bones, spinal cord problems such as injuries and compression, rheumatoid arthritis, and osteoporosis. These people should not take chiropractic medicine because it can cause more harm. The same applies to those using anticoagulants and antiplatelet. Chiropractic medicine may have negative effects on their condition.

- Other people who should be careful when taking chiropractic medicine are those suffering from cancer. Cancer patients are advised to consult a medical doctor before they start taking chiropractic medicine.

Meditation

Meditation is another form of alternative medicine which humans have been using for a long time. Although this method of healing has been around for many years, it is hard to tell when it began. Those who practice it will tell you that it probably started thousands of years ago. It's believed that meditation started during the prehistoric period. At that time, our ancestors would light up bonfires and stare at the flames. They basically engaged in some form of meditation by just staring at the fire. However, it was during the middle ages when the practice of meditation gained popularity in different parts of the world.

After many years, meditation started to become more influential. Just like many forms of alternative medicine, people from Asian countries like China, Japan, and India were among the first humans to experience the growing influence of meditation.

Religion is one of the main reasons why the practice of meditation was able to spread to many people across the globe. When we look at various belief systems, it is easy to notice that people who practice meditation are sometimes performing religious rituals. Different people in different parts of the world have their own belief systems that have influenced the practice of meditation.

If you look around, almost every religious group you know practices meditation in different ways. Religious groups also have different names for their type of meditation. In fact, people who practice the world's most popular religions like Christianity, Islam, Hinduism, Judaism, Buddhism, and Taoism practice meditation in various ways. You've probably seen people remain silent for a period of time at their places of worship for religious or spiritual reasons.

When it comes to meditation for healing purposes, this form of alternative medicine is often used to help people relax. Simply put, meditation is a relaxation exercise that is believed to have some health benefits. One of the best things about meditation is that it covers a wide range of dimensions. Most forms of alternative medicine and exercises only focus on the physical, mental, and emotional aspects of life. The practice of meditation covers these aspects as well as the spiritual dimension. Therefore, it is a good choice if you consider yourself to be a spiritual person.

Although many people engage in meditation to relax their body, this type of alternative medicine is more than a relaxation exercise. Its true essence is to help those who practice it to express their faith. Meditation allows you to build a strong relationship with whatever you believe in. This means that you can find your identity as a religious being and experience inner peace. In fact, meditation allows you to experience inner peace even if you are not a religious person because you get the opportunity to stay calm and contemplate in silence.

Benefits of Meditation

Of course, the main reason why you might consider using meditation is to capitalize on the benefits associated with this form of alternative medicine. The good news is that you can benefit from it in different ways. If you are ready to start your meditation sessions, you should be excited because meditation has the power to do the following:

- Reduce stress levels – meditation is a natural and healthy way to do away with any form of stress caused by challenging situations in your life
- Reduce the bad effects associated with aging
- Promote good mood
- Improve your ability to make good decisions

- Improve your ability to pay attention or concentrate
- Help the body grow healthy cells
- Change the way you think about life by promoting positive thinking
- Get rid of depression if you feel depressed
- Establish a good spiritual connection if you believe in the spiritual dimension of life
- Make you feel better and happier
- Improve brain functions including your cognitive abilities
- Improve a wide range of sleep problems including insomnia
- Improve your overall health by improving the functions of the body's immune system
- Improve metabolism
- Regulate emotions to help you achieve better control of your life

- Regulate breathing and improve the functions of the respiratory system by promoting healthy lungs

Clearly, meditation is one of the best forms of alternative medicine with a lot of benefits. Its benefits have made it a popular practice all over the world. Those willing to engage in meditation can expect to benefit physically, emotionally, mentally, and spiritually. Generally, there is an endless list of the good things that meditation can do for you. In addition to the health benefits associated with this practice, people who engage in meditation will tell you that it's one of the easiest forms of alternative medicine. It is accessible and you can do it without seeking help from another person.

Unlike other alternative treatments that require resources like needles, herbs, and spices, meditation does not require special tools. You only need yourself and a place where you feel comfortable. Another good thing about meditation is that it is not associated with some of the problems, side effects or adverse reactions you might experience when using other types of alternative medicine. Additionally, you don't have to spend money on meditation sessions.

Yoga

As we have seen in previous sections of this book, the Asian world has played an important role in inventing and popularizing different forms of alternative medicine. Yoga is another alternative treatment method that was first practiced in India. Just like meditation, this method of treatment focuses on all aspects of health including the physical, mental, spiritual, and emotional aspects. For this reason, it can be regarded as a holistic type of alternative medicine. The practice of yoga involves the use of a variety of religious beliefs from Buddhism, Hinduism, and Jainism.

It is said that yoga was first used during the Pre-Vedic Indian era. According to information from various texts, this practice emerged between the sixth and fifth BCE period. This was during the ancient Indian *Sramana* and *ascetic* movements. However, the practice remained unpopular until the twentieth century when it spread to the Western countries and other parts of the world. Clearly, yoga is an old practice and is now one of the most popular alternative treatment options.

One of the reasons why yoga has spread to many parts of the world and appealed to many people is its far-reaching religious range. It has reached many people leading to the establishment of various schools with the aim of teaching yoga to those interested in this kind of alternative medicine. However, it's important to keep in mind that the modern-day practice of yoga is not entirely influenced by traditional religious beliefs. Nowadays, the main goal of practicing yoga is to improve one's health and promote wellness.

Yoga is one of the practices that give interested people the opportunity to take part in classes. Today, you'll find yoga practitioners and enthusiasts in spas and clinics that promote and offer various yoga classes. If you've practiced yoga before, you probably know what a typical yoga class looks like. Just like an ordinary classroom with a teacher and students, yoga classes are composed of people who want to learn the practice and one or several instructors. The role of the instructor is to teach the students how to perform the various poses and postures in yoga. If you have never attended yoga classes, you should give them a try.

There are a number of important things to consider if you decide to practice yoga. First of all, it is advisable to meditate for a while before you start the actual exercise. In most cases, people who practice yoga usually spend about sixty to ninety minutes in yoga classes. Sometimes the classes may last for 2 hours depending on various factors. Regardless of how long you are going to do your chosen yoga exercises, it is important to start each session with meditation. We've already learned that meditation has the power to create a feeling of relaxation. If you start with meditation, you'll be able to clear your mind and get rid of any thoughts that may make it difficult to achieve inner peace during your yoga sessions.

Once you finish the meditation process, the next step is to start the actual exercise. You need to find something comfortable like a soft mat. To start your yoga session, lie down on the mat and try to control your breathing. The main purpose of regulating your breathing at this point is to ensure that you don't get tired easily during the session.

The practice of yoga encompasses a wide variety of movements and postures. Generally, it's up to you to choose the most appropriate posture for you. You may want to start with some common yoga exercises that are easy to perform even for someone who is doing yoga for the first time. One of the easiest yoga exercises involves lifting one leg. Once you lift your leg up, you are required to hold it in that position for a few seconds. The next step is to alternate the legs, lifting one at a time.

If you are satisfied with what you've achieved so far, you can move to other exercises such as the candle posture. This is a more challenging posture because you are required to raise both legs while standing on your shoulders with your buttocks in the air. You may also want to try other postures such as the prone posture and spine rotation.

One of the benefits of practicing yoga is the limitless freedom you get to experience during and after yoga sessions. It is a simple activity that can be performed by anyone. Additionally, you can engage in yoga any time you want and practice it regularly.

Yoga presents a number of benefits because of its power to influence different aspects of human health and life. As mentioned earlier in this section, yoga offers physical, mental, spiritual, and emotional benefits. Today, yoga is a widely used form of alternative medicine because of the fact that it can touch every aspect of human life. It's good for you if you want to improve your physical body shape, promote mental health, trigger good feelings, or get in touch with the spiritual world.

If you practice yoga on a regular basis, you will be able to:

- Improve your movement because yoga can make your joints more flexible
- Improve your posture with the help of the different postures
- Develop stronger bones that are healthy by doing a wide range of exercises
- Build up stronger muscular tissues
- Improve the health of your joints and the spine
- Develop stronger tendons and ligaments
- Improve the functions of the body's circulatory system

- Lower the risk of having injured joints and bones due to degenerative damage
- Boost your stamina so you can endure vigorous exercises
- Promote a feeling of balance
- Regulate the functions of various glands such as the adrenal glands
- Improve the activities of the body's immune system
- Sleep better than before
- Strengthen the heart to work better, especially its ability to contract
- Help the nervous system function better
- Prevent high blood pressure
- Improve your mood
- Lower your blood glucose levels
- Boost your ability to pay attention or concentrate
- Breathe easier because yoga exercises can expand your lungs
- Improve the functions of the digestive system

- Promote gastric motility
- Get rid of pains
- Improve your self-esteem and boost your confidence levels

You've probably noticed that yoga has one of the longest lists of benefits. This is enough evidence to prove that this type of alternative medicine has the power to change different aspects of your life. The good news is that all of the benefits listed here have enough evidence based on many scientific studies exploring the benefits of yoga. Many people from different parts of the world have chosen yoga because of the available evidence and the wide range of benefits they can derive from it. Perhaps it's time to start some yoga exercises if you haven't. Whether you are looking for physical, spiritual or emotional benefits, yoga is the right option for you.

It is normal for people who haven't tried something before to feel skeptical. If you still doubt the effectiveness of yoga, you need to do it yourself so you can learn from your own experience. As they say, experience is the best teacher. If you are just starting out and you don't know anything about the various postures, it is advisable to look for someone to guide you. Chances are you will find an instructor if you visit the nearest yoga spa where they offer yoga classes.

If you happen to have a good idea of what yoga entails and the various poses, then you can start your own yoga exercises at home. Create a yoga routine that best suits your daily schedule to avoid unnecessary inconveniences. You don't want to interfere with your work or home chores. If you need more information about yoga postures, you can read books or visit reliable websites. With the right sources of information, you will able to learn a wide variety of yoga steps, postures, and techniques that will promote your overall health and well-being.

Aromatherapy

Aromatherapy is another form of alternative medicine that has been around for hundreds of years. It is a holistic healing technique that involves the use of natural plant extracts to improve one's health and overall well-being. This method of healing is sometimes called essential oil therapy because it uses aromatic essential oils to promote healing on the physical, mental, and spiritual levels. Aromatherapy is both a science and an art that was developed by the ancient humans in different parts of the world including Egypt, India, and China.

Thousands of years ago, humans from the aforementioned regions and other parts of the world learned to incorporate aromatic plants components in oils, resins, and balms for religious and medical purposes. It's said that the famous French chemist René-Maurice Gattefossé coined the term "aromatherapy" in the 1920s. After doing research, he discovered the healing properties of certain essential oils and decided to classify plant essential oils based on their healing properties. Today, aromatherapy has gained popularity in the fields of medicine and science.

Aromatherapy uses one's sense of smell and skin absorption to improve the patient's health. It involves the use of various products such as diffusers, inhalers, facial steamers, cold and hot compresses, aromatic spritzers, body oils for topical application or massage, and clay masks. The most popular essential oils for aromatherapy include clary sage, fennel, eucalyptus, ginger, lavender, lemongrass, geranium, tea tree, rosemary, vetiver, Roman chamomile, patchouli, mandarin, helichrysum, and peppermint.

Benefits of Aromatherapy
Aromatherapy has a number of health benefits including the ability to:

- Treat a variety of conditions including asthma, fatigue, depression, insomnia, inflammation, arthritis, alopecia, menstrual problems, and erectile dysfunction
- Relieve pain
- Soothe sore joints
- Reduce stress and anxiety
- Treat migraines and headaches
- Ease labor discomforts
- Fight different types of virus, bacteria or fungus
- Reduce the side effects of chemotherapy
- Improve immunity and digestion
- Enhance sleep quality
- Uplift moods
- Manage cancer – aromatherapy massage is a popular complementary therapy for patients with cancer.

In addition to the above benefits, aromatherapy has gained popularity in healthcare settings as health practitioners try to use natural and effective methods to help patients. Some studies have proven that clinical aromatherapy programs reduce the need for expensive drugs prior to and after treatments. Hospitals and nursing homes are also making use of inhalation patches that allow patients to benefits from essential oils through inhalation. Generally, there's a considerable amount of evidence showing the benefits of the essential oils used in aromatherapy.

Drawbacks of Aromatherapy

- Essential oils are associated with a number of side effects including rashes on the skin, headaches, nausea, asthma attacks, and allergic reactions.

- Essential oils may not be good for persons with hay fever, asthma, eczema, epilepsy or hypertension. People with these health conditions should use aromatherapy with caution.

- Aromatherapy cannot replace professional medical attention if the patient shows clear signs of a medical condition. This form of alternative method should only be used to complement the body's immune system.

- Although research has proven the benefits of aromatherapy, scientific evidence is limited in certain areas. More research is needed to support the use of aromatherapy to treat persons with health problems like Alzheimer's disease and Parkinson's disease.

Homeopathy

Homeopathy is a pseudoscientific form of alternative medicine based on principles invented in 1796 by a German physician named Christian Friedrich Samuel Hahnemann. The term "homeopathy" is derived from the Greek words "Homeo" and "pathos", meaning "similar" and "suffering" respectively. The key thesis of this method of treatment is that a sick person can be cured using a substance that can produce the same symptoms like the ones exhibited by the patient when introduced to a healthy person's body.

Hahnemann conducted experiments using cinchona, a type of tree used to treat malaria. After ingesting the bark of the tree, he experienced the same symptoms as a person suffering from malaria. He then concluded that treatment could be done through similarity. According to him and the supporters of homeopathy, treatments must produce symptoms in healthy peoples similar to those of patients with the disease that needs to be treated.

Homeopathy's key premise is that each individual has a form of energy known as a self-healing response. Health problems occur when one's energy is messed up or imbalanced. Homeopathy works by stimulating the body's own healing responses.

Today, homeopathy is one of the largest forms of alternative medicine in the world with remedies derived from a wide range of natural substances from plants, animals, and minerals. Homeopathic medicines are available in different forms such as liquids, tablets, granules, and powder. Homeopathy practitioners consider the patient's physical, emotional, and mental symptoms in order to develop an effective treatment plan.

Benefits of Homeopathy

- Individuals using homeopathy do so to prevent and treat a number of health problems including depression, allergies, migraines, injuries, chronic fatigue syndrome, nausea, bruises, colds, coughs, toothaches, headaches, and rheumatoid arthritis.

- Homeopathic remedies are generally considered to be safe because they often contain water or alcohol with no serious side effects.

Drawbacks of Homeopathy

- The effectiveness of homeopathy has been disputed in medical science because some homeopathic preparations contain highly diluted substances that may have no healing effects on the patient.

- Controlled clinical trials have produced contradicting results regarding the effectiveness of homeopathy in treating certain health problems.

- Homeopathy cannot be used as a replacement for conventional care if the patient exhibits clear symptoms of a serious medical problem. You cannot use it for health-threatening diseases such as heart disease, cancer, and asthma.

Ayurveda

Ayurveda is one of the oldest forms of alternative medicine developed in India thousands of years ago. This medical system is based on ancient practices that involve the use of a holistic and natural approach to mental and physical health. Ayurvedic medicine is a combination of plant and animal products, minerals, metals, exercise, lifestyle, and diet.

The practice of Ayurveda is based on the belief that an individual's overall wellbeing depends on a balance between the body, mind, and spirit. A person is said to have good health if these three aspects are in harmony. Overall, the main objective of Ayurveda is to promote good health as opposed to fighting diseases. According to people who practice Ayurveda, every person's life revolves around five basic elements or *bhutas*, which include earth, water, space, air, and fire.

Benefits of Ayurveda

- A few studies have proven that Ayurvedic preparations may help manage symptoms in people with type 2 diabetes and reduce pain in persons with osteoarthritis.

- Ayurvedic preparations often contain turmeric, an herb that may help patients suffering from ulcerative colitis.

Drawbacks of Ayurveda

- Just like some other types of alternative medicine, there is insufficient scientific evidence to prove that Ayurveda can cure certain health problems. There is little scientific evidence based on a small number of clinical trials.

- Some Ayurvedic preparations contain potentially harmful ingredients. Therefore, it's important to check the ingredients all the time.

Reiki

Reiki is a form of alternative medicine that was first practiced by the Japanese before it spread to the Western world and other parts of the world in the 1970s. It was developed in 1922 by a Japanese Buddhist named Mikao Usui. The term Reiki consists of the Japanese words "Rei" and "Ki", which refer to "God's wisdom or the Higher Power" and "life force energy" respectively.

Reiki is basically an energy healing and spiritual technique that brings about healing on spiritual, mental, physical, and emotional levels. It mainly uses a technique known as hands-on-healing or palm healing to transfer universal energy from the practitioner's arms to the patient in order to encourage healing. Although Reiki is spiritual in nature, it's important to keep in mind that it's not a religion. You are not required to believe in any spiritual being to learn how to use and benefit from Reiki. It's all about laying hands on

68

a sick person to transfer and encourage the flow of "life force energy", which decreases when one is sick.

Just like other traditional forms of alternative medicine used in Asian countries, Reiki is believed to cause healing by controlling the body's flow of energy or *chi*. According to Reiki teachings, practitioners can manipulate an individual's *chi* to treat certain health problems. Medical research has not proven the existence of *chi* and that is why Reiki is considered to be a type of pseudoscience based on metaphysical concepts.

Reiki teachings also claim that we cannot exhaust the "universal life force energy" used for healing purposes. People who believe in Reiki say that anyone can access this energy through a process known as attunement. During this process, a Reiki master helps the student tap into the endless supply of "life force energy" to induce healing and improve the quality of one's life.

Benefits of Reiki

- Adherents of Reiki believe that the practice can influence the whole person including the body, mind, emotions, and spirit to bring health benefits.
- Some of the beneficial effects of Reiki as described in many books and other texts include a feeling of deep relaxation, peace of mind, security, improved immunity, better sleep, spiritual growth, pain relief, energy blockage removal, energy flow adjustment, and toxin removal among others.
- Reiki is a simple and safe method of healing that can be practiced by anyone.

Drawbacks of Reiki

- The main drawback of Reiki is the fact that there is no sufficient research evidence to prove that this healing technique can effectively treat health problems.

- Some Reiki adherents might avoid clinically proven medicine for serious health problems in favor of unproven alternatives like Reiki.

- The Reiki Master must actually touch the student's energy field, which is hard to prove.

Conclusion

In this book, you've learned about the different types of alternative medicine and their benefits. According to the available evidence, we all have a wide range of alternative treatments to choose from depending on our preferences, doctors' recommendations, or where we come from. Most of the alternative medicine practices that were discussed here have existed for many years and can bring remedy to a variety of problems including physical, emotional, mental, and spiritual problems.

Practitioners in the modern healthcare industry have embraced alternative medicine because of its extensive benefits. Your doctor may simply decide to prescribe some herbal medicine or advise you to practice yoga depending on your health condition. Generally, there is an endless list of alternative medicine practices that can be combined with conventional treatments to attain the best results.

Alternative medicine also seems to have a great future in the healthcare industry for a number of reasons. Although some types of alternative medicine need more research to prove their benefits, there is sufficient evidence to prove the benefits of some of the widely used alternative treatments.

Some people are still skeptical about the effectiveness of some forms of alternative medicine, but the truth is that it can actually help improve certain health conditions, prevent ailments, and even cure some diseases. It would be good if further researches will be conducted to be able to provide more scientific evidence to clear any doubts and support alternative options that may seem moot.

The decision to use alternative medicine is generally a personal choice, especially if you are looking for a natural remedy for common ailments. Usually, doctors prescribe manufactured drugs that contain high amounts of chemicals that usually come with side effects. Some of these drugs may cause adverse reactions and other life-threatening effects when not taken properly. The best thing about natural remedies is that they usually don't cause any side effects or adverse reactions. So, if you don't want to experience the bad effects of chemical-based drugs, you should give herbs, acupuncture, yoga, meditation, and other types of alternative medicine discussed in this book a try.

As you choose your preferred alternative treatment method, keep in mind that every individual is different. Listen to your body and identify which treatment works for you. For common health problems, going natural or using alternative medicine can be good for you. But for more complicated or severe health problems it is recommended that you consult a health practitioner immediately to know which treatment is better suited for you.

Made in United States
Cleveland, OH
23 December 2024